First Edition:

London, United Kingdom 2020.

Content production: Vanessa Badhia Rojas

Design, layout and illustration: Zamira Ávila

ACKNOWLEDGEMENTS

This is a book made with love and dedication. First of all, I want to thank God, without him, none of this would have been possible. He gave me the strength when tiredness was stronger than me, and he gave me the faith to continue believing in myself. My special thanks to my family: to my husband Manuel for motivating me to write this book and despite being with my newborn baby, encouraging me to find the ideal space to write.

To my father, Frank, and our productive talks and useful life advice, where I have often taken pleasant refuge, and for creating in me this desire to improve my health from an early age.

To the Central University of Venezuela and all my teachers who trained me as a professional.

To all those entrepreneurs who fundamentally taught me that dreams with action are productive realities.

To my patients who allow me to work every day to enhance their health and improve lifestyle.

To all of you who spend your time reading this book and thank you very much for always joining me.

I would like to dedicate this book to a very special person who will not be able to read it since she is in heaven, but who would be very proud of my growth as a person and as a professional. I dedicate this book to you, Mother, who shines in heaven. I love you mom.

TABLE OF CONTENTS

INTRODUCTION

Surely you have already read and tried thousands of failed diets, which have gotten you nowhere, so you may feel that you have wasted your time on simple attempts. To achieve eating habits that adapt to our needs is very difficult, especially today, where beauty stereotypes are so extreme that they lead some people to devise crazy diets, that many times people follow to attain that beauty standard. However, reality and fantasy are two concepts that are not always written on the same page, especially since the same thing can have different meanings from person to person. Starting from this concept that becomes ambiguous, I would like to share with you my experience as a nutritionist and explain the reason why many diets are not successful in the short, medium, or long term. Also, I will tell you what you can do to achieve your goal effectively.

Often the only thing we need to start walking a path is a little push, but with this book, I seek to offer you more than just a little motivation, I propose to give you the necessary tools to take your diet to another level and succeed in eliminating your bad eating habits forever. In the past, just like you, I tried different diets, supplements, exercises and massages to lose weight, it was a long process, full of disappointments and many falls, but that same process led me to understand what my mistakes were. For that reason, in this book I will tell you everything based on my personal and professional experience, I will tell you about the arduous task that it was for me to lose weight effectively and how I was able to achieve my goals, despite the temptations, stumbles and difficulties.

This book will give you the benefit of reading a nutrition expert who experienced first-hand the struggle of being overweight. I will explain to you many of the basic concepts when starting a diet or nutritional plan, so you can better understand the process you will go through. I will also tell you about nutrients, their enormous importance in a healthy diet and their biochemical interaction, all this in a simple way. Finally, you will access to healthy, balanced and effective recipes that you can include in your lifestyle.

Remember: If you want it, you can and you will achieve it, you just need to decide to start that change you want to see in yourself today.

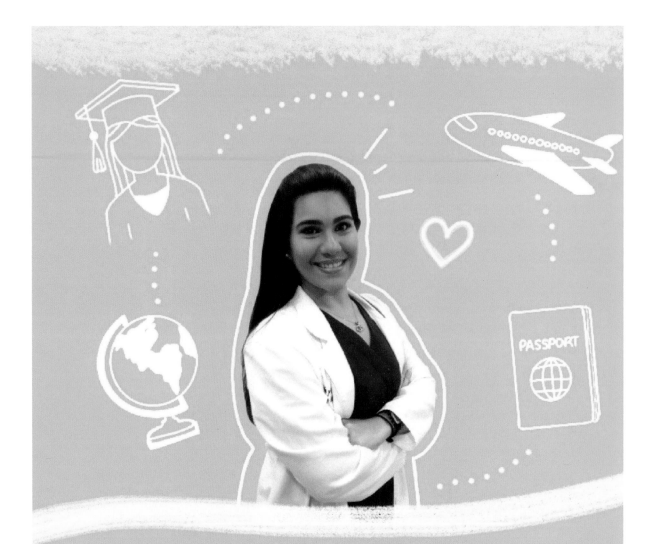

CHAPTER 1

MY STORY

CHAPTER 1

MY STORY

I would like to start this book by talking about how the change in my diet was.

It all started at the age of sixteen when I first visited a nutritionist. At that time, I was not aware of the health problems I had, nor of the long journey that I was starting, however, I clearly remember that when the nutritionist weighed me, the balance amounted to 100 Kg. At this moment, I only thought how difficult it would be to change my habits starting at home, which added to my clinical condition of polycystic ovaries and insulin resistance, it made the outlook seem hopeless.

My mother also had health problems associated with diabetes and hypertension, which is why my father, very concerned, decided to take the first step to help me improve my eating habits, motivating me every day and instilling in me a love for exercise and a healthier lifestyle.

I can proudly tell you that the first two months I managed to lose a total of 8 kg, which was a success for me. Then, when I graduated from high school something unexpected happened, I had the opportunity to enter one of the best universities in Venezuela, that is, the prestigious Central University of Venezuela(CUV), this event changed my life completely and I found myself very soon travelling to Caracas with four suitcases, where one of them was especially dedicated to food, once opened I could find biscuits, soft drinks, pasta, rice, canned food, in short, food of all kinds, especially high in sugar.

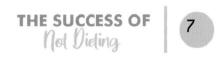

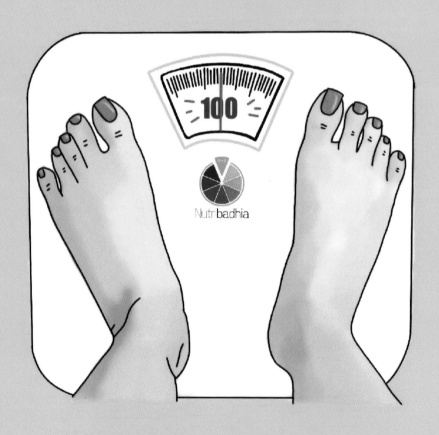

What do you think happened to all that food? Well, it took only a short time for the suitcase to be empty. In the evenings, feeling a little depressed and lonely, I would open my suitcases, grab anything and eat it together with my roommates. This cycle was repeated for many months. Not knowing how to cook food didn't help me much either, I clearly remember calling my mother on the second day of arrival, to ask her how to cook pasta. Thanks to that call, I learned to make pasta with margarine, a dish that became my main food for more than 3 months.

During that time, I was studying a degree in Biology at the CUV Faculty of Sciences. Over the months I gained not 10 Kg but 30 Kg, reaching 110 Kg. One day I sat down to cry in my room, I was very lonely and drowned in the food. I took a deep breath and thought: What are you doing, Vanessa? You cannot continue this way. This is your health; this is your well-being.

After this sad episode, I remembered that university enrolments would open in two weeks, and it occurred to me to study Nutrition and dietetics at the CUV I applied, I did it! I remember the night when the results were going to be published on the internet, I did not sleep thinking about whether that was my vocation. And after so many signs I was able to say: I DID IT!

I was already there, in the School of Nutrition and Dietetics of the Central University of Venezuela, to which I owe most of my knowledge. Studying this career made me change the way I saw eating, food and people who, like me, have suffered with weight and some clinical condition. Over the years during my degree, I was working on my diet, my body and my mind. I did not do it because of obsession, because —the truth should be told— many distrusted me, criticizing me, especially about the fact that an overweight or obese person could study nutrition. But this was my reason to show them that I could do it, and I lost around 30 Kg in 3 years, eating healthy without starving myself, and above all, exercising, because I like it, not because I had to.

So today, I want to thank everyone who was part of my change and I want to inspire anyone who believes that this is not possible to work hand in hand with me to guide them in a better lifestyle.

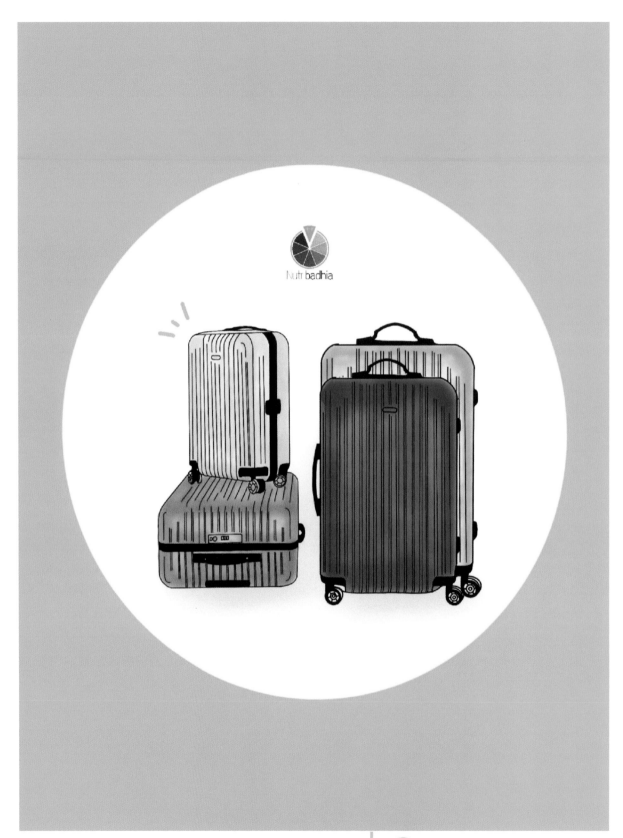

Upon graduating as a nutritionist, I started working in the area of clinical and aesthetic nutrition. Over the months I had an incredible opportunity to work in the sports area. During my experience in the area of nutrition, I attended many people with eating disorders, diabetes, obesity, hypo and hyperthyroidism, polycystic ovaries, among others, and I have realized that a large number of people needed nutritional education, because the first thing they begged for in the consultation was not to exclude certain foods from their diet, also naming amounts of diets that had not worked for them in the past. So, from that moment I decided to write this book.

Due to the situation in my country, Venezuela, I decided with my husband to emigrate to the United Kingdom, specifically London. During all that time, many things changed in my life and the way I perceived my surroundings. The first thing I wanted to do was validate my degree, but I wasn't sure if that was possible. Like all of us who emigrate, this is a great concern, so I decided to investigate and gradually collect the necessary documents and take the tests to validate my university degree. Two years later, I managed to validate in the UK, so now I am working as a Diabetes Specialist Dietitian. In addition to continuing with my international online nutrition consultation. It has been a long path and many efforts that I had to make along the way, but it has all been worth it, so it is always important to work on ourselves, and sometimes to leave our comfort zone to achieve our goals.

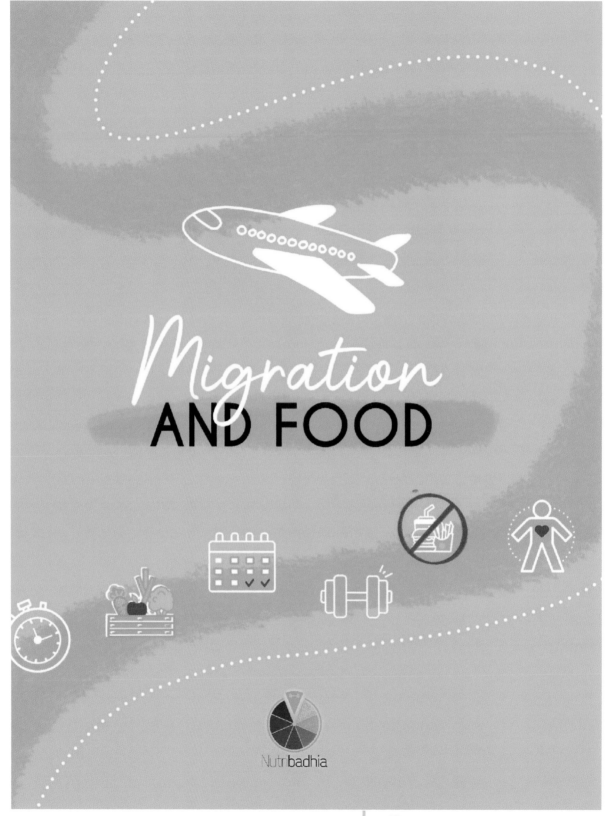

Migration
AND FOOD

MIGRATION AND FOOD

Emigrating made me change my routine and this had a great impact on my diet, therefore I would like to share some tips that I took in action after a period of adaptation. I have concluded that you should implement certain recommendations to prevent emigrating from affecting your health, especially your weight, and these recommendations are as follows:

- Take your time to adapt: one year at most for the adaptation period to work, routes, accessibility to food, mood, among others.

- Buy seasonal fruits and vegetables: the seasons are different in each country.

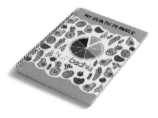

- Plan your meals, weekly purchases and workouts: This will help you meet any goal, but also create healthy lifestyle habits.

- Practice a sport or physical activity: to your preference, it doesn't have to be boring.

- Avoid temptations: do not buy anything that is not in your planning.

- Learn to know your body: This through your biotope, which I will explain later.

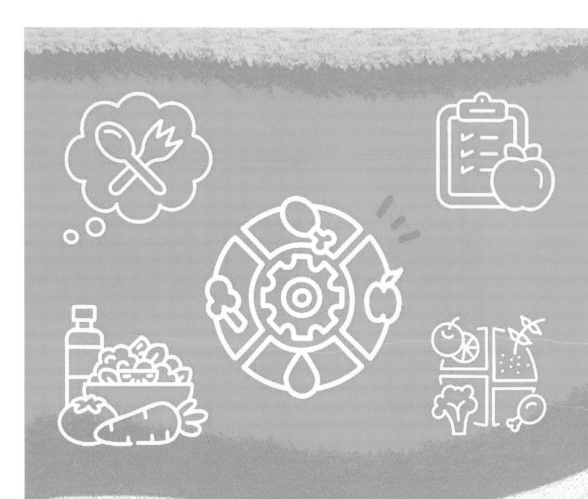

CHAPTER 2

BASIC CONCEPTS

CHAPTER 2

BASIC CONCEPTS

With my experience and everyday life I realized there is a lack of knowledge about the basic terms of nutrition, we tend to confuse a diet with a strict or restrictive diet, or we simply confuse hunger with anxiety, that is why I consider the importance of summarizing these basic concepts in this book.

Nutrition

Nutrition is the process by which the body ingests, digests, absorbs, transports, uses and excretes food substances, which allows the growth, maintenance and repair of the body. Except for food intake, the rest of the process is involuntary.

Eating

Eating is a voluntary process, by which the individual chooses the foods to be eaten according to their availability, tastes, habits and needs. It depends on social, economic, psychological and geographic factors, although this last factor is less distinctive in the developed world due to the possibility of transporting foods that can preserve their organoleptic and nutritional characteristics in a short time between different continents.

Foods

Foods, according to the Spanish Food Code, are «All substances or products of any nature, solid or liquid, natural or processed, which due to their characteristics, applications, components, preparation and state of preservation are likely to be habitually and suitably used for the normal human nutrition, such as fruitive or as dietary products, in special cases of human food».

Nutrients

Nutrients are components of food from which the organism is capable of performing the functions of growth, tissue repair and reproduction and can produce movement, heat or any other form of energy, as well as regulate these functions. They are classified according to the quantity present in the body, it is chemical composition, essentiality (impossibility of being synthesized by the human body) and function.

Diet

It is a set of food substances that a living being consumes regularly. This may or may not be healthy.

Metabolism

Chemical changes that occur in a cell or organism. These changes produce the energy and materials that cells, and organisms need to grow, reproduce, and stay healthy. The metabolism also helps to eliminate toxic substances.

Hunger

Physiological need to eat. Also is considered as a natural need to supply the body with food, produced by substances that operate at the level of the brain, in the hypothalamus; what happens about every 4 hours.

Appetite

Desire to eat a certain food. Appetite exists in all higher life forms and serves to regulate the adequate intake of energy to maintain metabolic needs.

The supply of nutrients must be carried out in such quantities that the following purposes are achieved:

o   Avoid nutrient deficiency.

o   Avoid excess.

o   Maintain the proper weight.

o   Prevent the appearance of diseases related to nutrition.

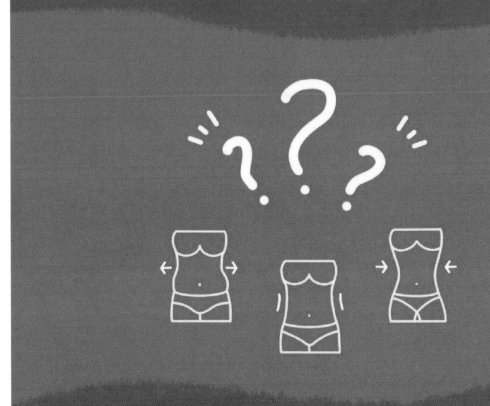

CHAPTER 3

KNOW YOUR BODY AND BODY COMPOSITION

CHAPTER 3

KNOW YOUR BODY AND BODY COMPOSITION

The first thing I would like to explain to you is that you, me, or anyone else can improve or harm the potential to burn fat, but you cannot change your genetics.

In the world of sports nutrition, there is another vision different from clinical nutrition. In both, body composition is important for making a nutritional diagnosis and achieving a goal, whether it is weight or health, so it is important that you know the biotypes and thus you can identify with probably one or two of them.

Biotope refers to the use of Biology for the classification of the human body according to its shape and some characteristics of the organism (metabolism, body composition, among others). It was first used in 1940 by William Sheldon, to whom this classification is credited. Many will wonder how this affects or benefits; Well, I can tell you that knowing your biotype will help you learn a little more about your diet and type of training to achieve your goals. When I started working with biotypes, I could see better results in myself and my patients, and for this, it is extremely important to know the body composition. I do it using anthropometric measurements (ISAK).

There are three types of Biotypes, and although I believe that each body is a universe, we can include them in these three groups:

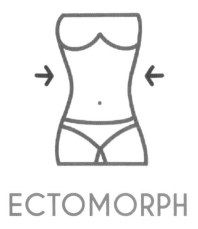

ECTOMORPH

They are people of slim build, low body fat, but also low muscle mass. They are characterized by having long muscles and very fast metabolism. The type of training recommended for ectomorphs is weight training, little cardio and a diet high in Complex Carbohydrates.

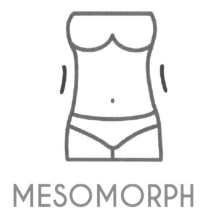

MESOMORPH

They are popularly known as 'standard'; these meet the best conditions for increasing muscle mass and decreasing body fat (yes, both at the same time, it is almost a miracle). They have an athletic bone structure and asymmetrical body composition. They have a regular metabolism and a V-shaped rib cage. The recommended workout is to alternate between cardio and weight training sessions at moderate intensity.

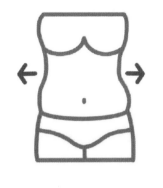

ENDOMORPH

They are people of robust build, they have a slow metabolism, they easily gain weight not only in muscle mass but also in body fat. The recommended diet for this Biotype is low in Carbohydrates (when I say low in Carbohydrates, I mean that it should always be in accordance with your daily requirements) and moderate fats. Training should be based on moderate-high intensity cardio and weight training. For this biotype, in particular, it is extremely important to calculate the caloric requirement according to the objective with a specialist.

Have you identified yourself with one yet?

Then let's leave some key points and let's get to practice!

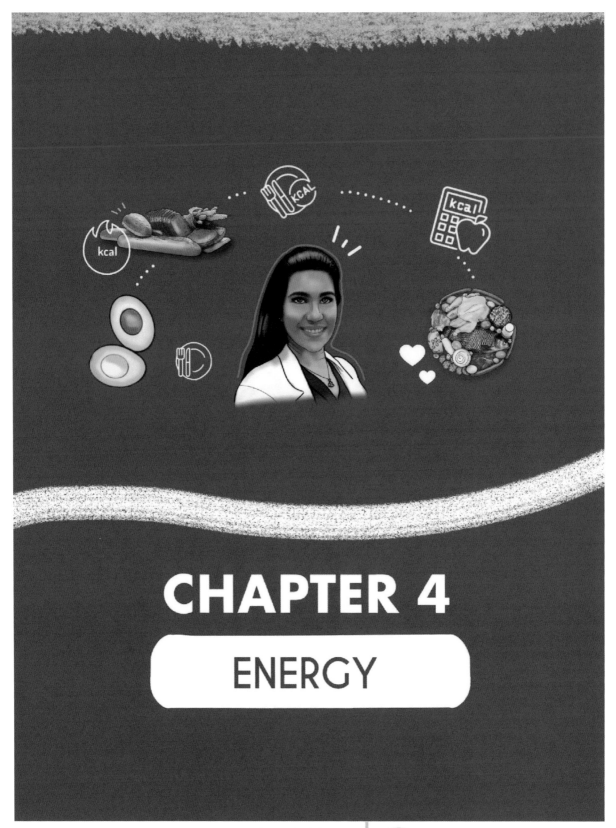

CHAPTER 4

ENERGY

CHAPTER 4

ENERGY

The functioning of the organism is possible thanks to various cellular metabolic processes. These involve the use of ingested nutrients and the disposal of waste products. In short, life is possible thanks to nutrition.

Obtaining energy for the body through macronutrients

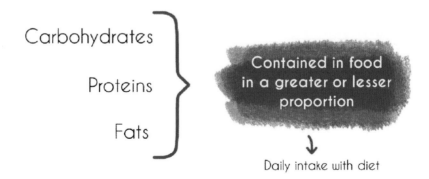

ENERGY UNITS

Food energy has been expressed in calories.

1 CALORIE =

amount needed to increase 1mg (1g) of water from 15.5°C to 16.5°C.

kcal

In nutrition, it is too small a unit, so the kilocalorie or Calorie is used. Currently also Joule.

Equivalences

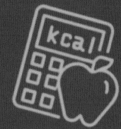

1 kcal = 1 Cal = 1000 Cal
1 kcal = 4,184 (4.2) kilojoules
1 kilojoule = 0.239 (0.24) kilocalories

The heat generated by the incineration or total oxidation of 1g of substance is called the caloric value or energy value of said substance. The ATWATER factor is used, which is the caloric heat that was assigned after making average estimates.

1g of carbohydrates ‑‑‑‑‑‑‑‑‑‑‑‑‑‑‑ 4kcal (16.8 Kj)
1g of protein ‑‑‑‑‑‑‑‑‑‑‑‑‑‑‑‑‑‑‑‑‑‑‑‑‑‑‑‑‑ 4 kcal (16.8 Kj)
1g of fat ‑‑‑‑‑‑‑‑‑‑‑‑‑‑‑‑‑‑‑‑‑‑‑‑‑‑‑‑‑‑‑‑‑‑‑‑‑ 9 kcal (37.8 kj)

The energy requirements of an individual are given by a series of factors: there are 3 main components that will define the energy needs for a given day:

1. Basal metabolism (what we should consume at least),
2. Physical activity,
3. Specific dynamic action (SDA) (also called Thermic effect of food (TEF) or dietary induced thermogenesis (DIT).

BASAL METABOLISM

It is the metabolic activity that is required for the maintenance of life and physiological functions in conditions of rest (not sleep). It is measured in:

● Full rest.
● Atmosphere with pleasant temperature.
● After the night fast.

This determination constitutes the basal metabolic rate (BMR), and we express it in kcal/kg/hour.

To calculate the BMR for the whole day:
♂ Male: 1kcal/kg/24 hours.
♀ Woman: 0.9kcal/kg/24 hours

Sleep:

During sleep the BMR decreases 10%. We can calculate the sleep rate (SR):

SR = 0.1kcal/kg/hour of sleep.

And we subtract this from the BMR

Most notable characteristics regarding basal metabolism:

- It is greater in men than in women.
- It decreases as age increases.
- It reaches the highest values during periods of rapid growth.
- Each individual has a practically constant basal metabolism.

Physical activity:

All physical activity increases energy requirements. To calculate what we are going to call activity rate (AR), we determine some standard values for different groups of activities:

Inactivity (little or no exercise) ---------------- Activity factor (1.2)

moderate activity (1-3 days per week) ------ Activity factor (1.375)

medium activity (3-5 days per week) -------- Activity factor (1.55)

high activity (6-7 days per week) ------------ Activity factor (1.725)

heavy activity (very hard exercise/more than 7 days per week) --- Activity factor (1.9)

Specific dynamic action (SDA) (or Dietary Induced Thermogenesis):

It refers to the energy that is put into play so that the processes of digestion, absorption, distribution and storage of the nutrients ingested with the diet take place, that is, the energy that is used as a supplement to convert the nutrients into organic components contained in the food eaten. We can calculate the specific dynamic action (SDA) as:

10% of the addition of BMR + AR

In summary, we could calculate THE ENERGY NEEDS OF AN INDIVIDUAL FOR A DAY as follows:

♂ Men: BM= IDEAL WEIGHT X 1 KCAL X 24 HOURS

♀ Women: BM= IDEAL WEIGHT X 0,95 KCAL X 24 HOURS

BMR corrected for hours of sleep:

BM corrected= Ideal weight x 0,1 Kcal x hours of sleep

BMR= BM- BM corrected

DCR (Daily calorie requirements) = BM corrected X Physical activity X SDA

For the ideal weight calculation, there are many formulas, however I like to use Mayo clinic, West:

♂ PI= Men: 22,1 x (height)2 (mts)

♀　　　 Women: 20,6 x (height)2 (mts)

Other factors that determine energy needs are:
- Growth.
- Weather.
- Thermoregulation.
- Psychic factors.
- Cultural factors.
- Age.
- Gender.

Energy balance and regulation

To maintain this balance there are two possibilities:

● Adjust the inputs to the outputs, that is, that the energy expenditure corresponds to the energy intake.

● Adjust the consumption to the inputs, that is, if the energy intake is higher than the expense, you must find a way to consume it, such as increasing physical activity on a regular basis.

This balance is regulated endogenously by neurovegetative and neuroendocrine factors and, thanks to the sensory input that connects with hypothalamic centres, food intake is regulated by feelings of hunger, thirst and satiety, among others.

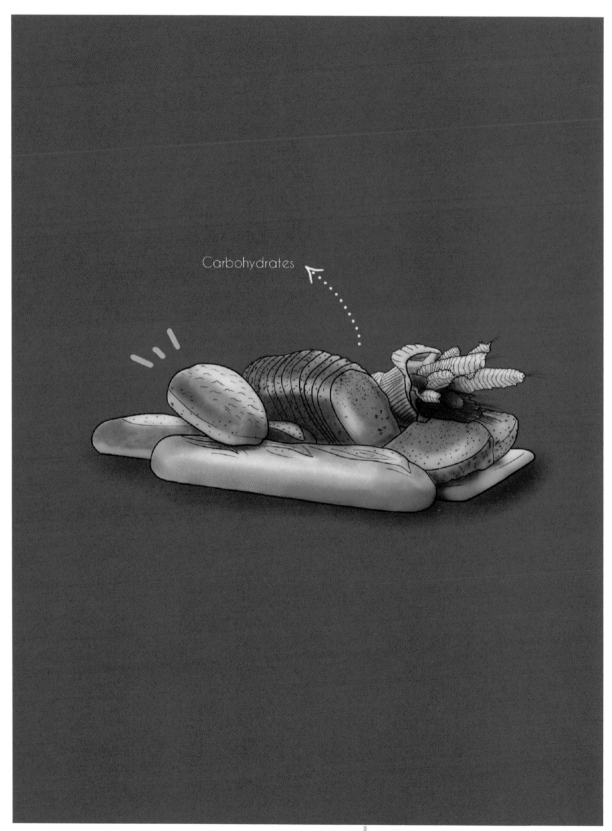

MACRONUTRIENTS

CARBONHYDRATES OR GLYCIDS

- Greater source of energy.
- Poor countries - diet with a high percentage of carbohydrates.
- Developed countries - diet with a low percentage of carbohydrates.
- They are found mostly in vegetables, fruits, and starches.
- In the form of glucose, it can be used by all cells without exception (brain).
- They are organic compounds formed by H, C and O.

CLASSIFICATION:

MONOSACCHARIDES

- Simple sugars.
- They cannot be unfolded by hydrolysis.
- Hexoses: 6 carbon atoms.

HEXOSES:

GLUCOSE (DEXTROSE)

- Grape sugar.
- Component of all disaccharides.
- Polysaccharide basic structural unit.
- It is also found in animal's blood.
- It is the only carbohydrate in the free state, all the rest are converted to glucose (liver).

FRUCTOSE (LEVULOSE)

- Sugar in the fruits.
- It is the structural unit of inulin (polysaccharide of certain roots and bulbs).
- It is very soluble in water.
- The most soluble of sugars.
- Widely used in diabetic diets (Does not require insulin to enter the cell).

GALACTOSE

- Lactose component produced during digestion.
- It is carried in the blood.
- It is obtained from the lactose disaccharide (milk).
- Less soluble than glucose.

SUGAR ALCOHOLS

SORBITOL - same caloric value as glucose.

MANITOL - half caloric value than glucose.

XYLITOL - it is used in chewing gums and does not cause cavities.

ETHANOL- it is obtained by fermentation of glucose. The larger the amounts of alcohol, the greater the total energy contribution.

1g of alcohol - 7-8kcal (but empty calories).

EVALUATION OF THE ABSORBED AMOUNT OF ALCOHOL

The following formula gives us the amount of alcohol consumed in grams based on the volume absorbed:

$$\frac{\text{Alcohol x density (0.8) x Volume (in cl)}}{10}$$

Example:

¼ litre of wine (25 cl) of 11° provides:

$$\frac{11 \times 0.8 \times 25}{10} = 22g \text{ of pure alcohol.}$$

HOW TO CALCULATE THE ALCOHOLEMIA RATE

The Widmark formula allows calculating the blood alcohol level of a fasting person, one hour after the absorption of alcohol:

$$\frac{\text{Pure alcohol (in grams)}}{\text{Weight (in kg) x 0.6 for women}}$$

0.7 for man

OLIGOSACCHARIDES: It is the union of 2 to 10 monosaccharide molecules. Disaccharides are the most important in nutrition.

SACCHAROSE (fructose + glucose)
- Specific enzyme (sucrase).
- Sugarcane or beet sugar are an example.
- It is the sweetest and cheapest way to take sugar.
- It is very soluble.
- It is found in many fruits and vegetables.

MALTOSE (glucose + glucose)

- Malt sugar.
- Specific enzyme (maltase).
- It is not naturally found in nature.
- It is made from starch by hydrolysis (in the process of digestion).
- It is less sweet than sucrose and more soluble.

LACTOSE (glucose + galactose)

- Specific enzyme (lactase).
- It is not of plant origin.
- It is not very soluble, not very sweet.
- It forms only in the mammary glands of lactating females.
- Fermented milk - yoghurt. Part of the lactose is converted to lactic acid.
- It is used in the manufacture of children's products and as an excipient in the manufacture of drugs.

POLYSACCHARIDES: complex carbohydrates.

Types of polysaccharides:

- Energy usable or digested.
- Not energy usable (dietary or dietary fibre).

STARCH

- Most abundant carbohydrates in our diet.
- Can be found in Cereal grains, tubers, legumes.
- To be able to be used (grinding or cooking).

GLYCOGEN

- Reserve of animal origin.
- It is stored in the liver and muscle.
- Can be found in Oyster and mussel, rich in glycogen.
- In many foods (storage and cooking), the nutritional value is nil.

CELLULOSE

- Main component of the wall of plant cells
- It is not digestible by animals; however, it is important to include it in the human diet (dietary fibre) because when mixed with faeces, it facilitates digestion and defecation, as well as prevents gases.
- It is found in sunflower seeds, corn, oats, among other carbohydrates with fibre.

HEMICELLULOSE

- Xylose polymer, arabinose and other monosaccharides
- They constitute the cell walls of fruits, stems and grain shells.
- They are not digestible, but they can be fermented by yeasts and bacteria.

PECTIN

- Derived from galactose
- It is found mainly in the skin of fruits and is used for the preparation of jams.
- It is very soluble in water and binds with sugar and fruit acids to form a gel.

AGAR

- Composed of galactose.
- When dissolved in water at high temperatures for subsequent cooling, it acquires a gelatinous consistency.
- It is used to thicken gastronomic preparations and to rinse beer.

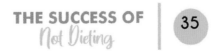

GUM

- Viscous vegetable exudates that segregate certain plant species to cover and close a wound.
- These exudates, when air-dried, become crystalline, translucent and brittle masses that dissolved in water serve as glue.

MUCOPOLISACARIDES

- They constitute the basic intercellular substance of the connective tissue.
- Examples are hyaluronic acid, which forms a sticky coating on some pathogenic bacteria.

FUNCTIONS OF GLYCIDS

1.   Energy supply

- Glycogenesis: glycogenic function or glycogen-making function from glucose
- Glycogenolysis: glycemic function or glucose-making function from glycogen.

2.   Energy storage:

Starch is the main store of sugars in plants and constitutes an important food for animals. Glycogen is the reserve of sugars in animals.

3.   Structural component:

Cellulose is the structural component of the walls of plant cells.

FOOD SOURCES

- Cereals: Rice, wheat, corn, barley, rye, oats, and millet found in starchy foods like bread, rice, pasta, breakfast cereals.

- Sugars: They are the second source of carbohydrates; they are obtained from sugar cane and beets. They are present in sugar, honey, jam, sweets.

- Tubers: The most consumed is the potato, 75% of its composition is starch but also contains simple sugars. In addition, the sweet potato, cassava, plantain, among others.

- Pulses: Chickpeas, lentils, beans, peas, soy. They are high in carbohydrates (50-55%).

- Fruits and vegetables: Although its carbohydrate content is lower than the previous ones.

PROBLEMS LINKED WITH THE CONSUMPTION OF GLYCIDS:

- Intolerances: malabsorption of different carbohydrates. Example: lactose intolerance, or other intestinal diseases.

- Carbohydrates and diabetes: an increase in the consumption of sucrose, an increase in weight, obesity, and a risk factor for type II diabetes.

- Carbohydrates and increased triglycerides: when the consumption of carbohydrates + alcohol increases.

- Carbohydrates and dental caries: sucrose increase + predisposingfactors.

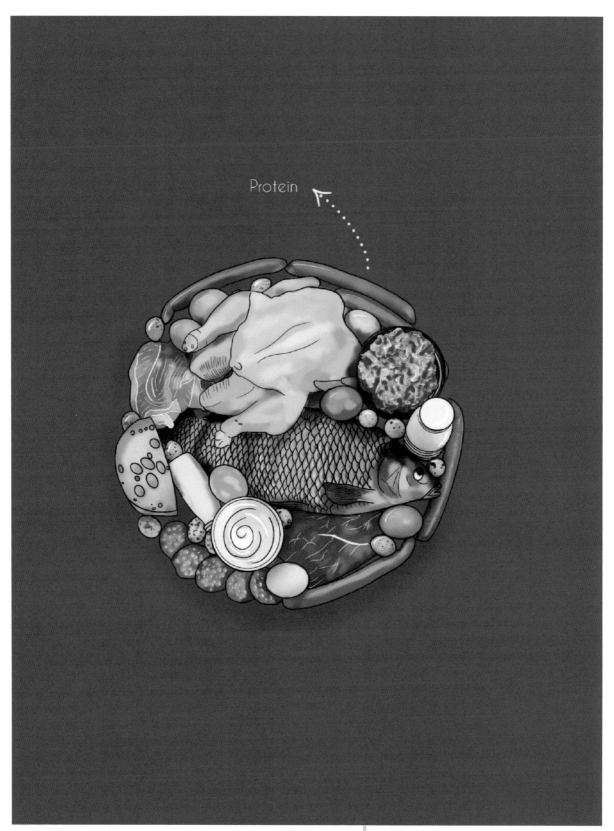

PROTEINS

They are the essential training element of all body cells. If there is an excess of protein, they are stored as an «energy pool». The body depends on the proteins in food. The quality and quantity of these compounds are of essential importance. The term protein - from the Greek "protos", which means first. In developing countries, there is low consumption of protein, especially of good quality. Therefore, the height of the population groups can be altered.

They are composed of C, H, O and N (some sulphur and phosphorous). They are formed from substances called amino acids, which contain nitrogen. Joined together by chemical ligatures, called polypeptide bonds. Peptides, polypeptides and proteins (the number of existing proteins can become infinite) are broken down by hydrolysis.

AMINO ACIDS

The amino acids that contain the body proteins are 20, and we classify them in:

- Essential: the body cannot produce it, we have to take them, and these are: isoleucine, leucine, lysine, methionine, phenylalanine, threonine, tryptophan, valine, histidine and arginine. The child does not produce Histidine, it must be provided with the diet.
- Non-essential: produced by the body and these are: alanine, asparagine. Aspartic acid, glutamine, tyrosine, cysteine, glycine, proline, serine and glutamic acid.

FOOD SOURCES

- **Food of animal origin:** They are high in protein and contain essential amino acids. They are meat, fish, eggs, milk and derivatives.
- **Vegetarian food:** They have protein and not all essential amino acids. They are cereals and derivatives, fruits, vegetables, and also legumes.

PROTEIN QUALITY OF THE DIET

Not only the quantity is important, but the quality, meaning, the amino acid profile that this protein presents.

Biological value (BV) measures the incorporation of amino acids from the diet into body structures. Food therefore has a different quantity and protein quality.

- Animal sources + legumes - greater Biological value
- Cereals and other vegetables - lower Biological value

PROTEIN COMPLEMENTATION

- Combination of two foods to achieve a protein of higher quality: Animal products (except eggs) and legumes are somewhat deficient in methionine. Starchy carbohydrate and other vegetables are very low in lysine (relative to methionine) (low Biological Value).

- The combination of both increases the quality of the protein (legumes + starchy carbohydrates):

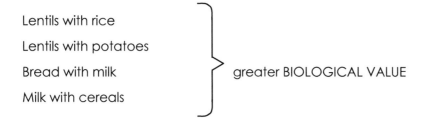

Lentils with rice
Lentils with potatoes
Bread with milk
Milk with cereals

} greater BIOLOGICAL VALUE

Complementation must be done in the meal itself.

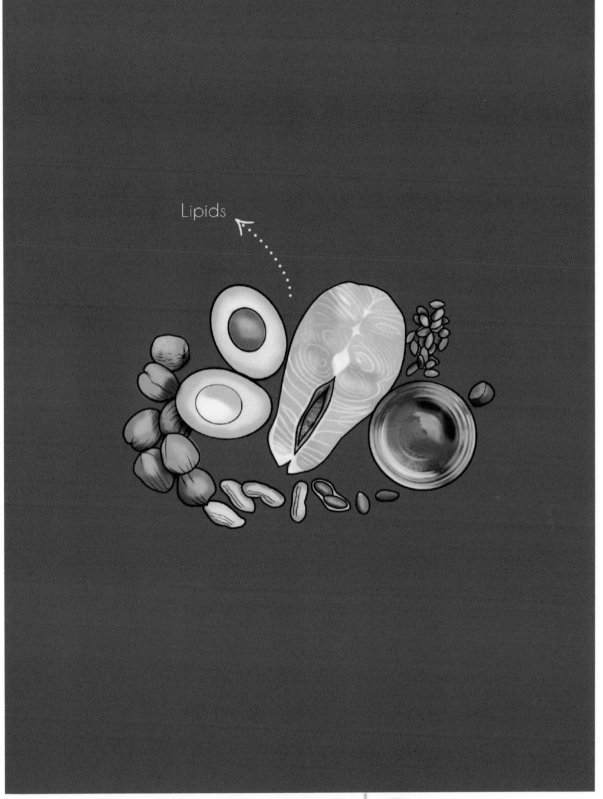

Lipids

LIPIDS OR FATS

Set of compounds of some heterogeneity, but which share the common characteristic of being insoluble in water, but soluble in organic solvents (ether, chloroform).

CLASSIFICATION

Considered from the food point of view:
- Triglycerides.
- Phospholipids.
- Cholesterol.

TRIGLYCERIDES

They are acylglycerols, a type of lipid, formed by a glycerol molecule, which has its three hydroxyl groups esterified by three fatty acids, saturated or unsaturated. Triglycerides are part of fats, especially of animal origin. The oils are triglycerides in a liquid state of vegetable origin or that come from fish.

Triglycerides are the main type of fat transported by the body. It receives the name of its chemical structure. After eating, the body digests fats from food and releases triglycerides into the blood. These are transported throughout the body for energy or to be stored as fat. Glycerol has 3 fatty acids in its structure.

PHOSPHOLIPIDS

They are amphipathic lipids, which are found in all cell membranes, and are arranged as lipid bilayers. They belong to the group of lipids derived from glycerol, presenting a structure similar to that of triglycerides. The current interest in them derives in their efficacy to incorporate different fatty acids at the cell membrane level since they have better absorption and use than triglycerides.

FATTY ACIDS

From a chemical point of view: they are straight chains of hydrocarbons that end in a carboxyl group at one end and in a methyl group at the other. There are 24 common fatty acids that differ in chain length and in the degree and nature of saturation.

Fatty acids are to be classified into:

- **Saturated Fatty Acids:** Those in which your carbon atoms have all the places saturated by hydrogen atoms. They are mainly concentrated in foods of animal origin (beef, chicken, pork) and plant products (coconut and palm oil).

- **Monounsaturated fatty acids:** they contain only one double bond (2 H atoms are missing). The main representative is olive oil (oleic acid). Also, peanut oil, almond, avocado, canola oil, sesame oil and others.

- **Polyunsaturated fatty acids:** those that have two or more double bonds (more than 2 carbon atoms have unsaturated places). The predominant in our diet is linoleic acid (it is contained in the main vegetable oils: sunflower oil. Coconut and palm acids have very little linoleic acid.

There are two main Polyunsaturated fatty acids families:
- **Omega 3:** This fatty acid cannot be produced by the body; however, we can obtain it through our diet in the form of blue fish or vegetable oils.
- **Omega 6:** This fatty acid is found in fatty foods or the skin of animals.

These families are not interchangeable and have very different biochemical roles.

CHOLESTEROL:

Cholesterol is one of the most important lipids or fats found in our body. It serves, fundamentally, for the formation of the membranes of the cells of our organs and as "raw material" for the synthesis of sex hormones and those of adrenal origin; It is also a precursor of bile acids, which are substances that are part of bile and that facilitate the digestion of fatty foods. In general, it is recommended not to ingest more than 300 mg/day.

Although cholesterol is a unique principle, as we have said before, it is transported in the blood by lipoproteins. Basically, there are two lipoproteins that are responsible for this transport: low-density lipoprotein (LDL) and high-density lipoprotein (HDL).

The former is responsible for bringing cholesterol to the tissues, and its excess is associated with the development of arteriosclerosis. HDLs remove excess cholesterol from cells and atheroma plaques.

In laboratory tests, in addition to total cholesterol, cholesterol linked to both types of lipoproteins is determined: LDL-cholesterol and HDL-cholesterol. Given their properties of increasing or decreasing atheroma plaques, they correspond to what is colloquially called "bad" or "good" cholesterol.

If you got here, you already know that the most important thing in nutrition is macronutrients, now I would like to explain the reason why I do not believe in extreme diets, and why they are not beneficial as long-term.

Reasons why you should avoid extreme low-calorie diets

Now, while we always end up with strict diets that in the long term only works to tell you what to do, I would like to list the reasons why you should avoid these strict/extreme diets, which from my perspective I find worrisome, especially looking at the number of people who come to me with clinical conditions, such as diabetes, that are a consequence of these diets.

- Diets increase hunger and cravings.
- Diets lower your metabolic rate.
- Diets can increase the risk of loss of muscle mass.
- Diets decrease the thermogenesis of activities that do not involve exercise.
- Diets decrease your ability to work and your activity.
- Diets decrease the functioning of your thyroid hormone.
- Diets lower the hormone leptin.
- Diets decrease the cortisol hormone.
- Diets lower testosterone.
- Diets increase weight gain.

Now that you know why strict diets are not a good idea, you will wonder what to do in order to lose weight, improve your skin, mood, improve your health in general. Don't worry, because here I have the answer:

Strategies to improve your body composition FOREVER without dieting and without getting depressed

- Think of it as a HABIT and not a DIET.
- Keep your muscle mass.
- Decrease calories moderately.
- Oxidize fat and don't store it.
- Caloric cycle (Do not stay with the caloric deficit for long).
- Lose weight at your RHYTHM.

The problem with perfection

Over time I understood that perfection doesn't exist, that it is just a bad concept that we have of ourselves, trying to compare ourselves with our friends, family and the entire social environment.

It has been very difficult for me not to worry about what people will say. Weight was always the most important thing in my life, until over the years I understood that this was not what I had to focus on, but on improving my health. My body will never be slim and that's something I understood.

I have been able to conclude that what I enjoy the most is exercising, this undoubtedly led me to achieve my health goal, but nowadays I see on social media the number of people who recommend eating less to avoid exercising, what do you think about this? Let's dig a little deeper ...

Exercise or eat less?

From my experience I have demonstrated that there are some reasons why exercise benefits more than reducing the calories and nutrients by half.

EXCERCISING (YOU OXIDIZE MORE)	DIET (EATS LESS)
Increase your metabolic rate.	Slow down your metabolic rate.
Create calorie deficit without triggering a hunger response.	Triggers the hunger response.
It provides many health benefits.	It can be harmful to your health in the long term.
Builds and helps maintain muscle mass.	It promotes muscle mass loss.
Increases hormones that have fat burning effect.	Decreases hormones that have a fat-burning effect.

CHANGE HOW YOU FEEL

If you could be in charge of how you feel it would be so much easier to eat better, I know. But I want you to know that how you feel affects your body, metabolism and energy levels, what you eat and how much exercise you will do. It is not a secret that when we are under stress situations losing weight is not easy nor healthy.

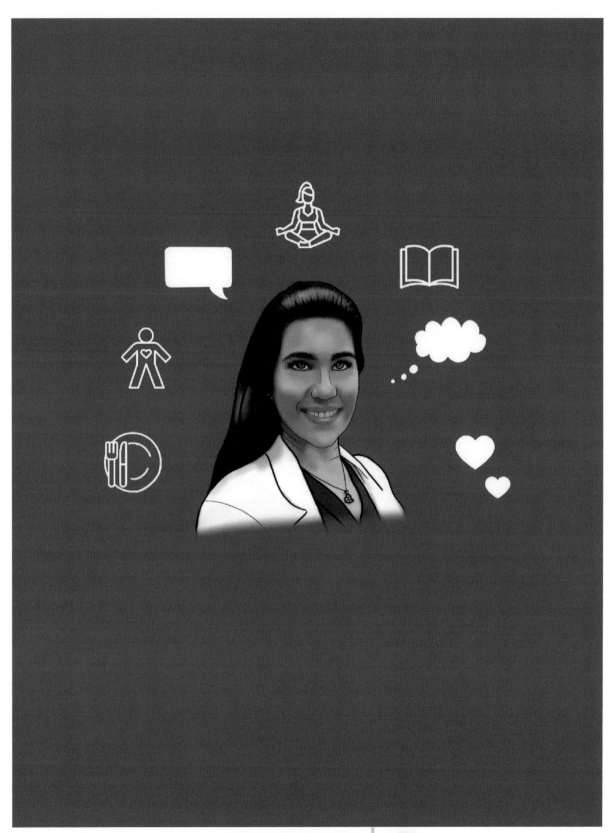

Mindfulness

Professor Mark Williams, former director of the Oxford Mindfulness Center, says mindfulness means knowing directly what is going on inside and outside of us, at every moment.

"It is easy to stop noticing the world around us. It's also easy to lose touch with how our bodies feel and end up living 'in our heads', trapped in our thoughts without stopping to notice how those thoughts are driving our thoughts, emotions and behaviour" he says.

Many times, we stop paying attention to what we do, what we eat and what we have around us. It is important to assess what affects, in this case, the time and type of food, as well as the place where we eat, since all this directly affects our relationship with food, in addition to adding stress and anxiety.

Since it is important for me to teach you how to have a better relationship with what you eat, let's play a game: according to the list that I will show you below, you must answer in each one the frequency with which you carry out that activity —Rare, sometimes, often - With this, you will be able to observe what aspects of your eating habits needs to be worked on.

List for eating consciously

I do the following:

- ☐ Eat until I'm fuller that I should.
- ☐ Eat until i'm full.
- ☐ Eat quickly, in less than 20 minutes.
- ☐ Eat while standing or while walking.
- ☐ Eat while driving.
- ☐ Eat when you are not hungry.
- ☐ Eat because the food is there.
- ☐ Eat while watching television.
- ☐ Eat in front of the computer.
- ☐ Wait while you are desperate or extremely hungry.
- ☐ Eat in response to stress or anxiety.
- ☐ Eat in response to depression or loneliness.

☐   Eat in response to frustration or being upset.

☐   Eat in response to boredom.

☐   Eat fast food because of not planning beforehand.

☐   Eat only because others eat.

☐   Eat because the time says it is time to eat.

☐   Know that you are done when the plate is completely empty.

According to science, what you see is what you eat. A Cornell University study compared people who had a transparent bowl with another white bowl, both placed on the same desk. The candies in the transparent bowl were visible while in the white bowl they were not. People in the clear bowl ate 71% more candy than people in the white bowl.

If you do most of these activities sometimes or often, we should definitely work on how to improve your relationship with food. In my practice, I use Mindful eating or conscious eating techniques, and for that, it is important to organize and practice with this list.

Eating consciously implies consuming food in a balanced way, that is why I will tell you how to improve your brain function through food. I know that many times with day to day we lose concentration, memory and cognitive abilities, that is why I always emphasize the importance of good nutrition to nourish our brain.

Foods to improve brain function

Nowadays, many studies prove that we can improve and promote concentration, intelligence, being alert, and improving our mood, in short, our brain function through certain foods that are very important for me to mention, They are 20 foods rich in vitamins, minerals, antioxidants, good fats and that are easy to include daily, these are:

1. <u>Whole grains:</u> If you got this far you will know how important it is to consume carbohydrates, it's very important to pay attention to quality. These contain vitamin B6, B12, B9 (folic acid) and have a low glycemic index, that is, they take longer to be digested and release energy more slowly. In contrast, refined grains or flours have a high glycemic index, are rapidly absorbed and cause fluctuations in blood glucose levels.

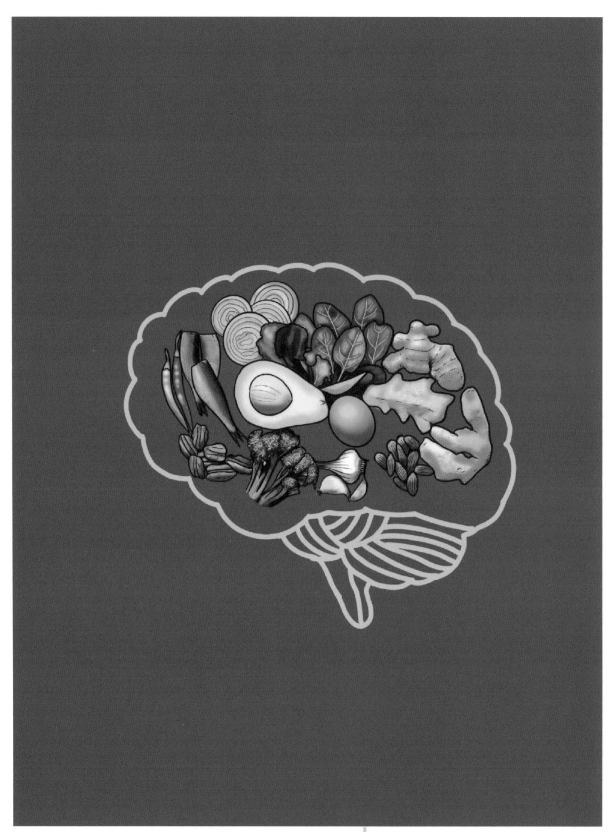

2. <u>Quinoa</u>: Quinoa and soy are considered the only vegetarian protein sources that contain all amino acids. Furthermore, it is high in fibre and phosphorous, magnesium, manganese, iron and copper, benefiting those who suffer from migraines.

3. <u>Walnuts</u>: They contain up to 20% of omega 3 and omega 6, essential fatty acids for healthy cell membranes in the brain, vitamin E and B6. They also help to maintain better levels of serotonin (neurotransmitter that influences our mood and appetite).

4. <u>Almonds</u>: Phenylalanine, is an essential amino acid in almonds that involves the production of adrenaline, norepinephrine, and dopamine. They are a source of vitamin E, riboflavin, iron, magnesium and L carnitine, which promotes the reduction of neuronal degeneration. It has also been shown to help lower "bad" LDL cholesterol while preserving "good" HDL.

5. <u>Cashew</u>: They increase the flow of oxygen in the brain, but it is also high in fibre, protein, iron, magnesium, phosphorous, zinc, manganese, polyunsaturated and monounsaturated fats. Something I love about cashews is that they increase serotonin levels.

6. <u>Pecan nuts</u>: A recent study shows that these nuts protect the brain from neuronal degeneration, but they are also rich in Vitamin A, B, E, folic acid, calcium, zinc, magnesium and phosphorus.

7. <u>Blackberries, blueberries, black currants</u>: Their main feature is their high levels of antioxidants and vitamin C that protect the brain from free radicals and oxidative stress that is involved in many of the clinical diseases. Furthermore, studies confirm that their consumption in combination with other good lifestyle habits protects against the diagnosis of cancer and heart disease due to its anthocyanin content.

8. <u>Strawberries</u>: They contain quercetin which inhibits the growth of cancer cells. In addition, it contains vitamin C which protects the immune system.

9. <u>Flax seeds</u>: Rich in omega 3 fatty acids, which help decrease stress, and some studies show that it improves postpartum depression, I noticed it in my personal experience. Furthermore, they are a source of fibre, folic acid, vitamin B6, manganese, magnesium, phosphorus and copper.

10. <u>Pumpkin seeds</u>: They have a high content of protein and fibre, magnesium, omega 6 and omega 3. I recommend adding these seeds in infant food since they also contain zinc which is usually deficient in children.

11. <u>Sunflower seeds</u>: They contain tryptophan, an amino acid that helps the brain make serotonin.

12. <u>Pomegranate</u>: High in antioxidants and folic acid, can be easily used for breakfast or snacks.

13. <u>Tomato</u>: High in lycopene, an antioxidant that contains different health benefits. These benefits are undoubtedly a protection against cardiovascular diseases, cancer and skin diseases. In addition, studies show that it improves memory.

14. <u>Broccoli</u>: Not everyone is aware of the calcium content of this vegetable, in addition to iron, vitamin K, which promotes memory and cognition.

15. <u>Avocado</u>: Known in other countries as avocado pear, and besides, it's my favourite fat, high in folic acid, healthy monounsaturated fats, which help maintain blood flow in the central nervous system, reduce blood pressure and improve the appearance of hair and skin.

16. <u>Wild salmon</u>: Perhaps it is not the cheapest fish I know, but it is certainly an excellent source of omega 3, which protects the nerves from cell membranes and is also responsible for long-term memory in the hippocampus.

17. <u>Eggs</u>: They contain tryptophan, as I explained earlier it is an amino acid. It has anti-inflammatory properties and a lot of vitamins and minerals. There are still people who think eggs increase cholesterol, and on the contrary, it helps to improve the cholesterol profile. There are two antioxidants the egg yolk, lutein and zeaxanthin, which benefit from macular degeneration and cataracts.

18. <u>Garlic</u>: It is a good source of selenium and helps improve oxygen flow to the brain. Also, it helps reduce bad cholesterol and has an antioxidant effect.

19. <u>Green Tea</u>: Green tea has been shown to improve memory and jib. It contains caffeine so you have to be careful with the amounts if you are pregnant or lactating.

20. <u>Dark chocolate</u>: Contains Phenylalanine, which increases alertness and good mental state.

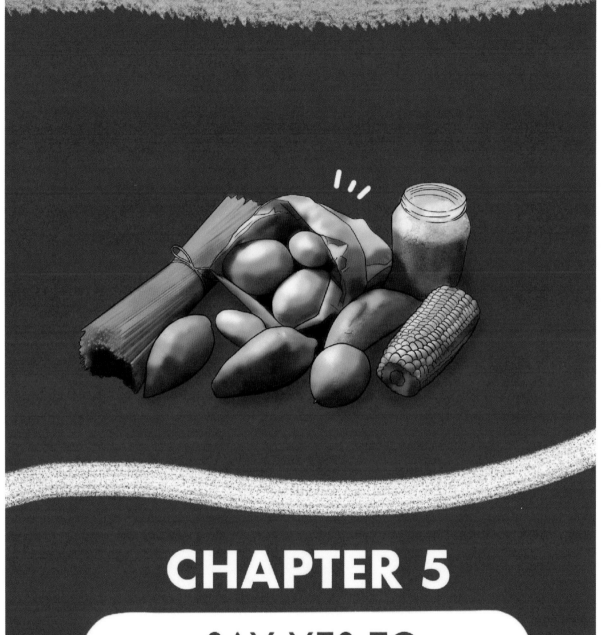

CHAPTER 5

¡SAY YES TO CARBOHYDRATES!

CHAPTER 5

¡SAY YES TO CARBOHYDRATES!

To conclude, in my last chapter of the book I would like us to take actions in your diet. If someone ever told you that you couldn't eat carbohydrates, forget it, don't listen to them! and wear your glasses so you can read me carefully. The term for this description is called Carbohydrate Cycle, from my experience, this is the best option for a healthy and lasting weight loss. I have more than 7 years using a carbohydrate cycle with myself and with many patients, and the results are brilliant in a long term. I am not saying that you cannot gain weight in the future, remember that our weight depends on many things, external, hormonal, environmental factors, among others, it would be very irresponsible of me to tell you otherwise. But I can assure that your carbohydrate anxiety and habits will improve a lot, you will not become stagnant, you will not change your mood, in short, you will feel much better without restrictions.

The carbohydrate cycle can be modified for Lean Muscle Gains or Fat Loss, as well as to maintain your weight. In simple terms, the carbohydrate cycle involves consuming a high amount of carbohydrates on some days of the week and a low to moderate amount of carbohydrates on other days. If you ask me, why not just go on a diet without carbohydrates? my answer would be that this triggers depression and low levels of thyroid hormone, which slows down your metabolism and on the 3rd or 5th day your body stops oxidizing fats.

High-carbohydrate days raise the body's insulin levels, fill glycogen stores, keep metabolism accelerated efficiently, and prevent muscle catabolism.

Low carb days are "fat burning days." Keep insulin levels low enough to allow maximum fat burning while maintaining muscle mass. For most individuals, this means having one or two high carbohydrate days per week which is a good starting point for fat loss.

In this book, I want to motivate and inspire you so you can do it, and if possible, the macro and micronutrients calculation should be done by a Nutritionist. Using the Carbohydrate Cycle methodology, I would like to present you with a scheme based on this program. You must know that it is only an example and that you should go to a nutritionist or dietitian for your personalized evaluation.

Monday	Tuesday	Wednesday	Thursday	Friday	Saturday	Sunday
Medium carbohydrate load	Low carbohydrate load	High carbohydrate load	Low carbohydrate load	Carga alta de carbohidratos	Low carbohydrate load	Low carbohydrate load

Remember that this scheme must always be monitored by a Nutritionist-Dietitian because the caloric calculation is what determines the weight loss and/or the increase in muscle mass in any diet or eating plan.

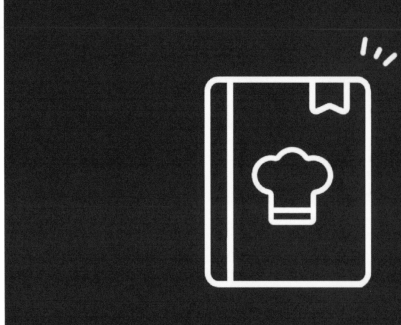

CHAPTER 6

RECIPES

CHAPTER 6

RECIPES

Now, theory

IS OVER

it's time to

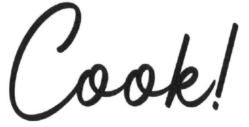

Cook!

BREAKFAST

1.   AVOCADO CREAM AND EGGS

Ingredients:

- 3 boiled eggs
- 1 small garlic clove, chopped
- 1 avocado, peeled
- 1 tablespoon of lemon juice
- 1 tablespoon of olive oil
- 3 tablespoons of coriander leaves, chopped

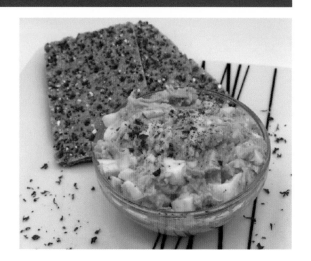

Preparation:

- Boil the eggs for 10 minutes, then pour cold water into the pot and let it cool.
- Once the shell has cooled, cut them into cubes and place them in a container.
- Crush the garlic and add it to the eggs.
- Remove the seed and skin of a half of an avocado and cut it into cubes.
- Place the avocado and coriander in the bowl. Drizzle with lemon juice and olive oil.
- Season everything with salt and pepper and mix gently. Garnish with more coriander.
- Serve immediately

BREAKFAST

2.   PANCAKES BASE

Ingredients:

- 1/3 cup oat flakes
- 2 whole eggs
- 1 tablespoon ground flaxseed
- Cinnamon and vanilla to taste
- 1 sachet of sweetener (Optional)

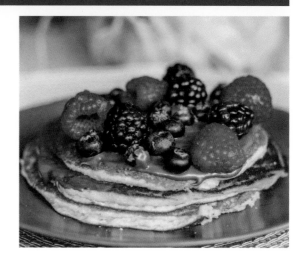

Preparation:

- Mix all the ingredients until you get a homogeneous mixture, then prepare the pancakes (3 small or 2 medium) in a non-stick frying pan, if necessary, you can spray in a little oil or with the help of a napkin.

- Pair them with fresh fruit or sugar-free jam. If you wish, you can add nut butter without added sugar or oils.

BREAKFAST

3.   OAT WAFFLE

Ingredients:

- 2 egg whites
- 3 tablespoons of oatmeal (or oat flakes blended)
- Pinch of baking powder
- Sweeten to taste
- Pinch of cinnamon powder
- 1/2 tablespoon of protein (optional)
- 1 glass of water or almond milk or skimmed milk

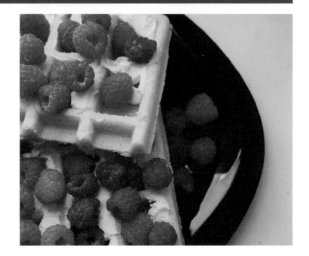

Preparation:

- First, you mix all the dry ingredients together, add the egg whites and stir, add a splash of water to taste and take it to the waffle maker or pan, without oil and at low heat so that it cooks well, flip for a few seconds and that's it.

- Accompany it with 1 teaspoon of peanut butter and 1 teaspoon of sugar- free marmalade or jam.

BREAKFAST

4.   COTTAGE CHEESE PANCAKES

Ingredients:

- 1 heaped cup (250 g) of cottage cheese
- 3 eggs
- 1 tablespoon of vanilla sugar
- 1 tablespoon of coconut sugar
- 3 tablespoons of oat flour or almond flour

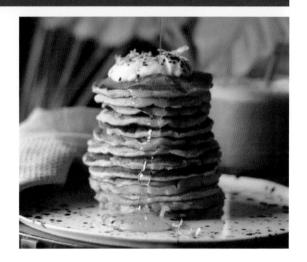

Preparation:

- Put the cottage cheese in a bowl, add the egg yolks (keep the whites separate) and mash everything with a fork. Add flour and mix well.

- Beat the egg whites until you have a stiff foam and add to the cheese mixture, gently combine the ingredients.

- Heat a dry, non-stick skillet and fry the pancakes (about 2 tablespoons of dough per pancake) in batches, for about 3 minutes, until the bottom is lightly browned. Flip and cook for another 2 minutes.

- Suggested portion: Greek yoghurt, and berries.

BREAKFAST

5.   FRENCH TOAST

Ingredients: (2 Toasts)

- 2 slices of whole wheat bread
- 1 egg
- 1/2 cup of almond milk (or whichever you use)
- 2 tablespoons of Whey Protein vanilla (optional)
- 1 teaspoon of cinnamon
- 1 teaspoon of stevia
- 1 teaspoon of butter (optional)
- Jam sugar-free

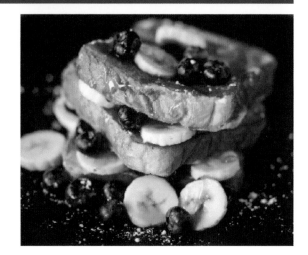

Preparation:

- Mix the milk, the egg, the stevia, the cinnamon, and the whey protein if you are going to use it, in a container. Heat a non-stick skillet and divide the teaspoon of butter into 2 portions. Soak the bread slices through the mixture. Add 1 of the butter portions to the pan. Add the bread in the pan on top of the butter and crush with a spatula.

- When It's brownish, flip the other side.

- Serve by placing the marmalade or jam sugar-free on top or low-fat cheese if you want.

LUNCH

1. SMOKED AUBERGINE GOULASH

Ingredients:

- 2 aubergine
- 2 tablespoons of olive oil
- 1 onion, diced
- 2 garlic cloves, minced
- 1 red bell pepper, chopped
- Juice of 1 lemon or lime
- Paprika to taste (Optional)
- 1 red chili, finely chopped

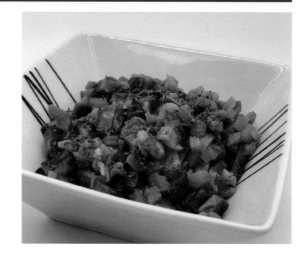

Preparation:

- Wash the aubergine and cut into ¼ inch slices. Season on both sides with salt and reserve for about 20-30 minutes, until the aubergine absorbs water.

- In a large saucepan, heat 1 tablespoon of olive oil and fry the onion for 2 minutes, then add the minced garlic and cook together for another 1-2 minutes. Add the chopped red pepper and finely chopped chillies. Cook for about 4 minutes, stirring constantly.

- Dry the aubergine with paper towels and cut into cubes. Add it to the pot and add 1 tablespoon of oil. Cook for approximately 10 minutes, meanwhile, mixes occasionally. While cooking, add lemon juice, season with paprika powder and freshly ground black pepper (you no longer need to add salt because the eggplant has already absorbed the salt).

LUNCH

2.   ZUCCHINI LASAGNE

Ingredients:

- 5 Courgettes
- Shredded chicken
- Peeled tomatoes
- Basil
- Sea salt

CAULIFLOWER BECHAMEL

- 1 large onion
- 150 grams of cauliflower
- Pinch of sea salt low in sodium
- Nutmeg powder
- Pepper
- 1 cup of Almond milk

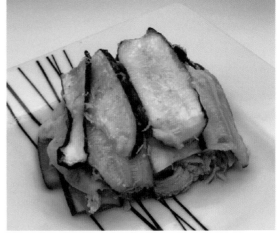

Preparation:

- Cut the courgettes into slices, season it with a pinch of sea salt and seal over a frying pan on both sides, so that later they release less water.

- You need some shredded chicken made with plenty of vegetables, peeled and crushed tomatoes, basil, a pinch of sea salt.

- In a previously greased saucepan, sauté the chopped or cut onion next to the

LUNCH

2.   ZUCCHINI LASAGNE

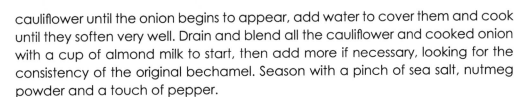

cauliflower until the onion begins to appear, add water to cover them and cook until they soften very well. Drain and blend all the cauliflower and cooked onion with a cup of almond milk to start, then add more if necessary, looking for the consistency of the original bechamel. Season with a pinch of sea salt, nutmeg powder and a touch of pepper.

- To assemble the lasagne, place a bit of cauliflower béchamel in the bottom of a container that you can take to the oven, then the slices of courgette, shredded chicken, low-fat or vegetable pasteurized cheese, some lean, low-fat ham, Then we finish with another layer of courgette slices, cauliflower béchamel sauce and low-fat cheese. Bake until gratin and ready.

- Remember that this sauce can be used as a complement for any type of vegetables and whatever you want.

LUNCH

3.   SOUP WITH SHRIMPS

Ingredients:

- 4 cups (1lt) vegetable stock
- 2 tablespoons (30 g) of tomato paste
- 1/2 cup (100 ml) canned coconut milk
- 1 cup (225 g) canned, chopped tomatoes
- 1 cup (100 g) shiitake mushrooms, chopped
- 3/4 cup (200 g) shrimp
- 2 tablespoons of fish sauce
- 1 tablespoon of lime juice
- Coriander, for garnish
- Chilli, to decorate

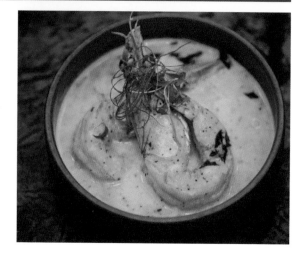

Preparation:

- Pour the vegetable stock into a pot, add the tomato paste and boil.
- Add coconut milk, tomatoes and mushrooms, cook for about 5 minutes.
- Then add the shrimp and cook for about 1 minute over low heat. Season with fish sauce and lemon juice.
- Garnish with fresh coriander and chilli.

LUNCH

4.   QUINOA WITH VEGETABLES

Ingredients:

- 1 cup of raw Quinoa
- Vegetables stock
- Chives
- Sweet pepper
- Garlic
- Mushrooms
- Peppers
- Capers
- Broccoli
- Carrots
- Rosemary
- Balsamic
- 1 Tablespoon of olive oil

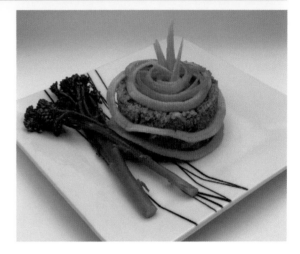

Preparation:

- To prepare the quinoa I use a cup which I previously washed very well with a splash of water. Then, I place it with two cups of water in a pot.

- I use vegetable stock and cook over low heat covered until done. Then I add chives, sweet pepper, garlic, mushrooms, paprika and capers.

- Serve with steamed broccoli and baked carrots with rosemary and balsamic.

LUNCH

5.   RICE WITH CHICKEN AND DRIED TOMATOES

Ingredients:

- 2 clean chicken breasts, cut into pieces
- 1 paprika
- 1 onion
- 3 sweet peppers
- 3 garlic cloves
- 1 teaspoon of olive oil
- 5 slices of dried tomato
- 1 teaspoonful of oregano
- 1 stalk of chives
- 1 tablespoon of turmeric
- 1 tomato
- Salt and pepper
- 2 cups of brown rice
- 4 cups defatted chicken broth or water
- Parsley to taste
- 1 bay leaf

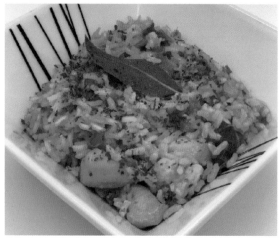

LUNCH

5.   RICE WITH CHICKEN AND DRIED TOMATOES

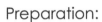

Preparation:

- Season the chicken with garlic, oregano, salt and pepper and marinate for two hours. Place the olive oil in a saucepan and sauté the onion, paprika, sweet pepper and chives, all minced. Add the chicken and sauté well.

- Add the tomato and the dried tomato. Wash the rice and add it. Add the water or broth, the turmeric and the bay leaf. Check the salt and cook over low heat for 40 minutes.

- Serve by sprinkling with parsley. Enjoy and bon appetit!

DINNER

1. SPINACH WRAP

Ingredients:

- 1/2 cup rolled oats
- 1 tsp ground flaxseed
- 1 handful of spinach leaves
- Pinch of nutmeg powder
- Garlic powder
- 3 egg whites plus 1 yolk
- No more than 1/4 cup of a splash of water or almond milk

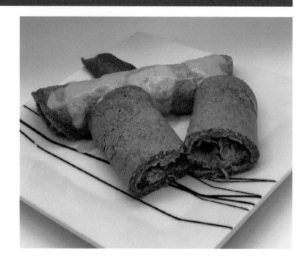

Preparation:

- Add everything in the blender until it's very well blended; it should be a semi-liquid mixture, let it rest for a minute while you heat the pan, then we cook it in a previously greased non-stick frying pan, we flip it as soon as it rises up around the edges and we leave it there a little more and that's it.

- I stuffed them with shredded chicken, tomatoes, lettuce and a mustard tip.

DINNER

2.   TUNA NUGGETS

Ingredients:

- 1 cup of tuna
- 1/2 chopped onion
- 1 egg
- 1 handful of chopped spinach
- 2 tablespoons ground flaxseed
- Salt to taste

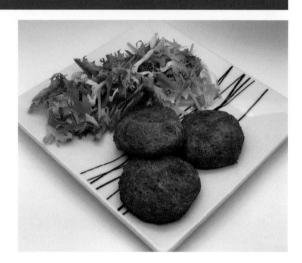

Preparation:

- Mix all the ingredients very well and put together the nuggets. Place them in frying pan or Airfryer until cooked and browned on both sides.

- You can bake them on a tray approximately 20 minutes until browning. Accompany with a delicious salad.

DINNER

3.   ROASTED TUNA FILET WITH CITRUS VINAIGRETTE AND BASIL AROMA

Ingredients:

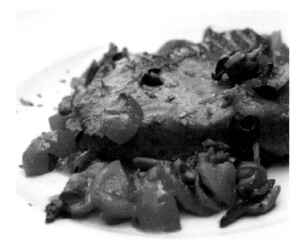

- 1 piece of tuna loin (500 g).
- 3 tablespoons of soy sauce.
- 3 tablespoons of lemon juice.
- 1 green lemon.
- 1 orange.
- 4 cherry tomatoes.
- 1 fresh chive.
- A few basil leaves.
- 8 tablespoons of olive oil.
- Salt.

Preparation:

- Mix the soy sauce, lemon juice, orange juice and olive oil. Macerate the tuna for about 20 minutes in this mixture. Roast the tuna piece with the marinade in the oven at medium temperature (180°) for 15 minutes.

- Save the juices from the roast for later use. In a frying pan, make a sauté with the julienned chives (thin strips), the tomatoes and the basil leaves.

- Cut the tuna filet into slices and accompany it with the roast juices and the cocktail tomatoes with the basil aroma. Sprinkle the preparation with a little green lemon zest.

- Sprinkle the mixture with a little green lemon zest.

DINNER

4.   SALMON SPRING ROLLS

Ingredients:

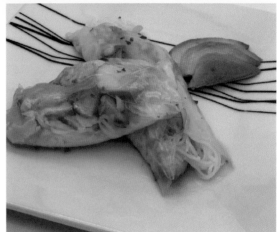

- 4 sheets of rice paper
- Fresh coriander
- 7 oz. (200 g) salmon, cut into 4 pieces
- 1 tablespoon of coconut oil
- Soy sauce or tamari for serving

Preparation:

- Boil a little water in a frying pan, remove from the heat and immerse in the rice paper one after the other, soak for 30 seconds. Remove the sheets from the water and place them on a damp cloth.

- Place a piece of coriander on each leaf, top with a piece of salmon, sprinkle with freshly ground black pepper, and wrap the rice paper around the fish.

- Heat the oil in the pan and fry the rolls for 2 minutes, then flip and cook for another 2 - 2.5 minutes until golden brown.

- Put on a paper towel, cool slightly and serve with soy sauce. Perfect with a salad.

DINNER

5. CHICKEN THIGHS WITH RICE IN SAUCE

Ingredients:

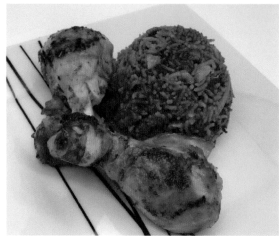

- 2 tablespoons of coconut oil
- 8 skinless chicken thighs
- 1 cup (200 g) of Basmati Rice
- 4 chopped chives
- 4 garlic cloves, sliced
- 1/3 cup (200 ml) of white wine
- 2 heaped cups (500 ml)
  Chicken soup
- 4 tablespoons dried blueberries

For the sauce:

- 3 tablespoons soy sauce
- 2 tablespoons of rice vinegar
- 1 tablespoon of peanut butter
- 1 teaspoon of chili flakes
- 1 teaspoon of honey
- 1 teaspoon of sesame oil

DINNER

5. CHICKEN THIGHS WITH RICE IN SAUCE

Preparation:

- Heat oven to 375 °F (190 °C). Heat the oil in a large skillet.
- Season the chicken thighs with salt and pepper and cover them for 5 minutes on each side until golden brown, then remove from heat and transfer to a plate.
- Pour most of the fat from the pan, leaving about 1 tablespoon in the pan.
- Add the peeled and sliced garlic and the tender onion, fry for 1 minute in the skillet.
- Add uncooked rice and fry again for about 1 minute. Pour in the wine and cook for another 2 minutes until most of the liquid evaporates.
- Then add all the ingredients for the hoisin sauce, the hot broth and the blueberries, boil it.
- Transfer the rice to an excess-proof dish and place the chicken thighs in the centre. Bake in the preheated oven for 30 minutes.
- Once cooked, divide it into 4 dishes and serve, or store in the refrigerator for up to 2-3 days.

HEALTHY DRESSINGS

PASSION FRUIT DRESSING

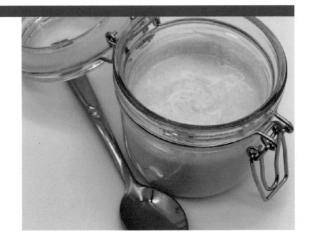

Ingredients:

- 1 cup natural yogurt (No sugar added)
- ¼ cup of passion fruit juice
- 4 teaspoons olive oil
- Sweetener to taste
- Salt and pepper to taste

Preparation:

Gently mix the yogurt with the oil and then the passion fruit juice, add the sweetener and season to taste.

MANGO DRESSING

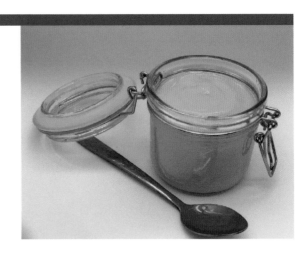

Ingredients:

- 1 medium ripe mango
- ½ cup of fresh lemon juice
- 3 tablespoons of olive oil
- 1/8 teaspoon crushed red pepper
- Salt and pepper to taste

Preparation:

Chop the mango into cubes and take it to the blender with the lemon juice until you get a puree-like consistency. Transfer the mixture to a bowl and beat with the olive oil. Finally, add salt and pepper to taste.

HEALTHY DRESSINGS

ORANGE DRESSING

Ingredients:

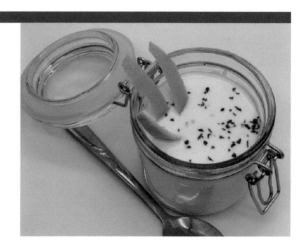

- 1 cup natural yogurt (No sugar added)
- ¼ cup of passion fruit juice
- 4 teaspoons olive oil
- Sweetener to taste
- Salt and pepper to taste

Preparation:

Combine all ingredients in a bowl and season to taste.

STRAWBERRY DRESSING

Ingredients:

- 1 cup of natural yogurt (No sugar added)
- 1 cup fresh strawberries
- 1 tablespoon red wine vinegar
- Sweetener to taste

Preparation:

Blend all ingredients until it's a smooth mixture.

HEALTHY DRESSINGS

BASIL DRESSING

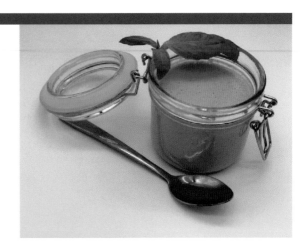

Ingredients:

- ½ cup natural yogurt (No sugar added)
- 10 gr of basil
- 1 bit of chives
- 4 teaspoons olive oil
- 6 teaspoon apple cider vinegar
- 1 clove garlic, minced
- Salt and pepper to taste

Preparation:

Put all the ingredients in a blender until you get a smooth cream. Finally, add salt and pepper to taste.

MAYONNAISE DIET

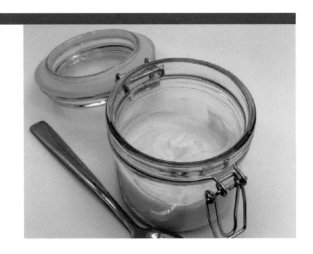

Ingredients:

- 200 gr of cottage cheese
- 2 teaspoon mustard
- Juice of 1 lemon
- Salt to taste

Preparation:

Mix all the ingredients until obtaining a homogeneous mixture.

HEALTHY ALCOHOLIC BEVERAGES

These alcoholic beverages should be taken with awareness and, less frequently, despite being healthy they contain calories, so my recommendation is to consume them 1 time a week.

Cheers!

TEQUILA SUNRISE

Ingredients:

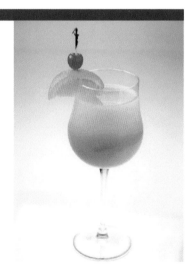

- 50 ml of Tequila
- 1 Natural orange juice
- Cranberry juice (without sugar)
- Ice

Preparation:

1. In a glass with ice, combine the tequila with the orange juice.
2. Cover with the cranberry juice.

HEALTHY ALCOHOLIC BEVERAGES

CLASSIC MOJITO

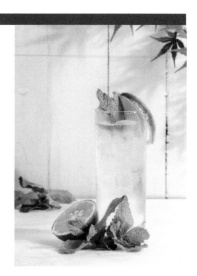

Ingredients:

- 12 fresh mint leaves
- ½ lemon juice
- 1 Tablespoon of agave
- 1 ½ ounces white rum
- ¾ cup of mineral water
- Lemon slice for garnish
- Fresh or frozen fruit (Strawberry, blueberry, mango or kiwi)
- Ice

Preparation:

* In case it is a fruit mojito add the fresh or frozen fruit of your choice at the bottom of the glass at the beginning.

1. Add 12 fresh mint leaves, lemon and agave to a glass.
2. Add ice and rum along with mineral water.
3. Garnish with the lemon wedge.

HEALTHY ALCOHOLIC BEVERAGES

BLOODY MARY

Ingredients:

- ¾ cup low-sodium tomato juice, unsweetened
- Juice of ½ lemon
- 100 ml vodka
- Hot sauce
- Worcestershire sauce
- Freshly ground pepper
- Ice
- 1 lemon wedge and celery to garnish

Preparation:

1. In a glass mix the tomato juice, lemon, hot sauce, Worcestershire sauce and pepper.
2. Add ice and vodka.
3. Garnish with a lemon wedge and celery.

HEALTHY ALCOHOLIC BEVERAGES

VODKA RICKEY'S

Ingredients:

- 1 tablespoon of agave juice of ½ lemon
- 2/3 oz of a digestive liquor (Campari, Cynar, etc.)
- 1 cup of mineral water
- Ice

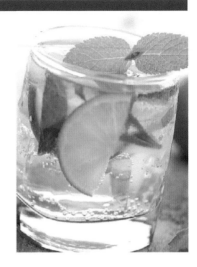

Preparation:

1. In a glass with ice, combine the lemon juice, agave and liquor.
2. Cover with mineral water.

HEALTHY ALCOHOLIC BEVERAGES

SEA BREEZE

Ingredients:

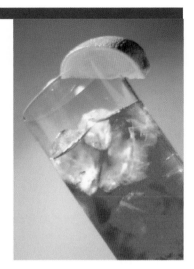

- 1 oz cranberry juice with no added sugar.
- 1 drop of grapefruit juice
- 1 oz vodka
- Ice
- Mineral water

Preparation:

1. Place the vodka and the cranberry juice in a glass.
2. Add the grapefruit juice.
3. Place in a glass with ice.
4. Add a splash of mineral water.

BIBLIOGRAPHY

1. British Dietetic Association. (2020). Obtenido de British Dietetic Association: https://www.bda.uk.com/

2. Deirdre K tobias, M. C. (2020). National Library of Medicine. Obtenido de Effect of low-fat diet interventions versus other diet interventions on long-term weight change in adults: a systematic review and meta-analysis: https://pubmed.ncbi.nlm.nih.gov/26527511/

3. Elsevier. (2020). Elsevier. Obtenido de Elsevier: https://www.elsevier.es/

4. Food and Agriculture Organization of the United Nations. (2020). Obtenido de FAO: http://www.fao.org/home/en/

5. Instituto Nacional de Cancer. (s.f.).

6. Lauren Owen, B. c. (2020). National Library of Medicine. Obtenido de The rol of diet and nutrition on mental health and wellbeing: https://pubmed.ncbi.nlm.nih.gov/28707609/

7. Metabolismo. (2020). Obtenido de Instituto Nacional de Cancer: https://www.cancer.gov/espanol/publicaciones/dictionary/def/metabolismo

8. well, E. (2020). nhs Live well. Obtenido de nhs UK: https://www.nhs.uk/live-well/eat-well/starchy-foods-and-carbohydrates/

9. (Food and Agriculture Organization of the United Nations, 2020) (Lauren Owen, 2020)